Fitness Revolution
Believe, Build, and Achieve Your Best Self

ANILA FERRERO

Printed in the United States of America

ISBN: 9798342025737

Disclaimer

This book is intended for informational purposes only and does not constitute professional advice. While the author has undertaken diligent efforts to ensure accuracy, there is no guarantee of accuracy or of no errors, omissions, or typographical errors.

The author is not liable for any financial, legal, or other consequences arising from the use of this book's material. Readers should consult a qualified professional before taking any action based on the information provided.

Dedication

To those who sought to break me: your shadows forged my resilience and redirected my path. To those who showed me kindness: your support lit the way. This journey embodies both. With gratitude.

Table of Contents

Preface

Welcome to the world of fitness—a realm where the journey to a healthier, stronger, and more vibrant version of yourself begins. If you're holding this book, chances are you're ready to take that first step or refine your existing routine. Either way, you're in the right place.

Fitness is more than just a series of workouts or a diet plan; it's a holistic approach to improving your overall well-being. In this book, we'll explore the fundamental topics that lay the groundwork for a successful fitness journey. My goal is to provide you with practical insights and actionable advice to help you navigate through the complexities of exercise, nutrition, and motivation.

We start with understanding the core types of exercise and techniques, ensuring you grasp the essentials of cardio, strength, flexibility, and balance. Each of these elements plays a crucial role in a well-rounded fitness routine and mastering them will empower you to create a balanced workout plan tailored to your goals.

Next, we dive into the art of crafting effective workout programs and planning. Developing a strategy that aligns with your personal objectives can be a game-changer. I'll guide you through the principles of progression, recovery, and variety, helping you design a program that maximizes results while keeping you engaged and motivated.

No fitness journey is complete without addressing nutrition and hydration. What you fuel your body with directly impacts your performance and recovery. We'll cover the basics of healthy eating, hydration strategies, and how to tailor your nutrition to support your fitness goals.

Injury prevention and management are also critical components of any fitness regimen. Understanding how to prevent common injuries and how to address them if they occur will ensure you stay on track and maintain your momentum. I'll provide practical advice on proper form, warm-up techniques, and effective recovery strategies.

Finally, we'll delve into the subject of motivation and mental health. The road to fitness is as much a mental challenge as it is a physical one. We'll discuss strategies to keep you motivated, overcome obstacles, and harness the positive effects of exercise on your mental well-being.

This book is a guide to transforming your approach to health and wellness. Whether you're starting from scratch or looking to refine your existing routine, my aim is to equip you with the knowledge and tools you need to succeed. Let's take that journey together.

Here's to your health, strength, and happiness.

Anila Ferrero

Introduction

Achieving a well-rounded fitness routine requires more than just understanding how to exercise; it involves integrating multiple aspects of health and wellness into your lifestyle. This book will provide you with the essential knowledge needed to build a comprehensive fitness plan that supports overall physical well-being.

Exercise Types and Techniques

- Understanding the different types of exercise (cardio, strength, flexibility, balance) and how to perform them correctly is fundamental. This knowledge helps in creating a balanced fitness routine that targets various aspects of physical health.

Workout Programs and Planning

- Designing an effective workout program involves knowing how to structure workouts for strength, endurance, and weight loss. It also requires incorporating principles like progression and recovery. A well-planned program maximizes results and minimizes the risk of overtraining or injury.

Nutrition and Hydration

- Proper nutrition and hydration are essential for supporting physical performance, recovery, and overall health. Understanding how to fuel the body with the right nutrients and fluids can enhance workout effectiveness and help achieve fitness goals.

Injury Prevention and Management

- Preventing and managing injuries is crucial for maintaining long-term fitness. This involves learning about proper exercise form, appropriate warm-up and cool-down practices, and how to address common injuries effectively.

Motivation and Mental Health

- Maintaining motivation and mental health is vital for long-term fitness success. Motivation, through intrinsic and extrinsic factors, helps overcome challenges and ensures consistency. Good mental health, supported by exercise, mindfulness, and self-care, enhances adherence. A positive mindset, including resilience and positive self-talk, sustains progress and commitment.

By exploring these essential components, you will be equipped to develop a fitness regimen that is both effective and sustainable. Let's dive in and embark on a journey towards better health and fitness together

Exercise Types and Techniques

An effective fitness routine encompasses a variety of exercise types, each contributing uniquely to overall physical health. Understanding the fundamental types of exercise—cardio, strength, flexibility, and balance—and how to perform them correctly is essential for building a well-rounded fitness program. Here's a brief overview of each exercise type and its role in creating a balanced fitness routine:

Cardio: The Heart of a Balanced Fitness Routine

Cardiovascular exercise, commonly known as cardio, is a cornerstone of a balanced fitness regimen. It encompasses a range of activities designed to increase your heart rate and improve the efficiency of your cardiovascular system. Understanding the various types of cardio and how to perform them correctly is crucial for achieving optimal health and fitness.

What is Cardio?

Cardio exercises are activities that elevate your heart rate and breathing, improving your heart and lung health. They include activities like running, cycling, swimming, and brisk walking. The primary goal of cardio is to enhance cardiovascular endurance, which is essential for overall fitness and well-being.

Types of Cardio Exercise

- **Steady-State Cardio**: This involves maintaining a consistent intensity throughout your workout. Activities like jogging or cycling at a moderate pace fall into this category. Steady-state cardio helps build endurance and is effective for burning calories over longer durations.
- **High-Intensity Interval Training (HIIT)**: HIIT alternates between short bursts of intense activity and periods of rest or lower intensity. For example, sprinting for 30 seconds followed by a minute of walking. HIIT is highly efficient for

improving cardiovascular fitness and can be completed in a shorter time compared to steady-state cardio.

o **Low-Impact Cardio**: Activities such as swimming, rowing, or using an elliptical machine are considered low-impact. They are gentler on the joints and are ideal for individuals with joint issues or those recovering from injury.

How to Perform Cardio Correctly

o **Warm-Up**: Always start with a warm-up to prepare your body for exercise. A 5-10 minute warm-up of light cardio, like brisk walking or gentle jogging, helps increase your heart rate gradually and reduces the risk of injury.

o **Maintain Proper Form**: Good form is essential for maximizing the effectiveness of your workout and preventing injury. For example, when running, ensure your posture is upright, and your stride is comfortable. In cycling, adjust the bike to the correct height to avoid strain.

o **Monitor Intensity**: Use tools like heart rate monitors or perceived exertion scales to gauge the intensity of your workout. Aim for a target heart rate that aligns with your fitness goals—whether that's fat burning, endurance, or peak performance.

o **Cool Down and Stretch**: After completing your cardio session, spend 5-10 minutes cooling down with light activity followed by stretching. This helps in gradually lowering your heart rate and aids in muscle recovery.

Incorporating Cardio into Your Routine

To achieve a balanced fitness routine, integrate cardio with other exercise types, such as strength training, flexibility exercises, and balance work. Aim for at least 150 minutes of moderate-intensity cardio or 75 minutes of vigorous-intensity cardio per week, as recommended by health guidelines. Vary your cardio activities to keep your routine engaging and to target different muscle groups.

Cardio exercise is vital for improving cardiovascular health, enhancing endurance, and supporting overall fitness. By understanding the different types of cardio and performing them correctly, you can build a well-rounded exercise routine that contributes to your long-term health and well-being.

Strength Training: Building a Strong Foundation

Strength training is a key component of a well-rounded fitness program, focusing on building muscle strength, endurance, and overall physical power. It involves exercises that challenge your muscles through resistance, enhancing not only muscular strength but also bone density and metabolic rate. Understanding the different types of strength training and how to perform them correctly is crucial for maximizing your results and maintaining a balanced fitness routine.

What is Strength Training?

Strength training exercises involve using resistance to induce muscle contraction, which builds strength, endurance, and muscle mass. Common forms of strength training include weight lifting, resistance band exercises, and bodyweight exercises like push-ups and squats. The primary goal is to improve muscle strength and functional fitness, which supports everyday activities and overall health.

Types of Strength Training

- **Free Weights**: Includes exercises using dumbbells, barbells, and kettlebells. These allow for a full range of motion and engage multiple muscle groups simultaneously. Examples include bench presses, deadlifts, and bicep curls.

- **Machine Weights**: Utilizes weight machines that guide your movements along a fixed path. These machines can help target specific muscle groups and are often easier to use for beginners. Examples include leg presses and chest fly machines.

- o **Bodyweight Exercises**: Uses your own body weight as resistance. These exercises can be done anywhere and are effective for building strength and endurance. Examples include push-ups, squats, and lunges.

- o **Resistance Bands**: Involves elastic bands that provide resistance during exercises. They are portable and versatile, suitable for both beginners and advanced exercisers. Examples include resistance band squats and shoulder presses.

How to Perform Strength Training Correctly

- o **Warm-Up**: Begin with a 5-10 minute warm-up, such as light cardio or dynamic stretching, to prepare your muscles and reduce the risk of injury.

- o **Maintain Proper Form**: Good form is essential for maximizing the effectiveness of your workout and preventing injury. For example, when performing a squat, keep your back straight and knees aligned with your toes.

- o **Progressive Overload**: Gradually increase the weight, resistance, or intensity of your exercises to continue challenging your muscles and promoting growth. This principle ensures continued progress and avoids plateaus.

- o **Cool Down and Stretch**: After your strength training session, spend 5-10 minutes cooling down with light activity followed by stretching to aid in muscle recovery and flexibility.

Incorporating Strength Training into Your Routine

To achieve a balanced fitness routine, combine strength training with cardio, flexibility exercises, and balance work. Aim for at least two non-consecutive days of strength training per week, focusing on different muscle groups each session. Vary your exercises and gradually increase the challenge to keep your workouts effective and engaging.

Strength training is crucial for building muscle, enhancing endurance, and supporting overall physical health. By understanding and correctly performing various strength exercises, you can develop a comprehensive fitness routine that contributes to long-term strength and well-being.

Flexibility Training: Enhancing Mobility and Range of Motion

Flexibility training is an essential aspect of a well-rounded fitness regimen, focusing on improving the range of motion of your muscles and joints. It involves exercises designed to stretch and lengthen muscles, enhancing overall mobility, reducing stiffness, and supporting functional movement. Understanding the different types of flexibility exercises and how to perform them correctly is vital for achieving a balanced and effective fitness routine.

What is Flexibility Training?

Flexibility training consists of exercises that increase the length and elasticity of muscles and connective tissues. This type of training helps improve joint range of motion, reduces muscle tension, and enhances overall physical performance. Common flexibility exercises include static stretching, dynamic stretching, and foam rolling. The primary goal is to enhance movement efficiency and reduce the risk of injuries.

Types of Flexibility Exercises

- o **Static Stretching**: Involves holding a stretch in a stationary position for a specific period, typically 15-60 seconds. This type of stretching helps lengthen muscles and improve overall flexibility. Examples include hamstring stretches and quadriceps stretches.

o **Dynamic Stretching**: Involves moving parts of your body through a full range of motion, often performed as part of a warm-up. Dynamic stretching prepares your muscles for exercise by increasing blood flow and mobility. Examples include leg swings and arm circles.

o **Foam Rolling**: Uses a foam roller to apply pressure to muscles and release tightness. This self-myofascial release technique helps improve flexibility and alleviate muscle soreness. Common foam rolling techniques target areas like the back, thighs, and calves.

o **PNF Stretching (Proprioceptive Neuromuscular Facilitation)**: Involves a combination of stretching and contracting muscles. Typically performed with a partner or trainer, this method helps achieve greater flexibility gains through alternating muscle contraction and relaxation.

How to Perform Flexibility Exercises Correctly

o **Warm-Up**: Start with a 5-10 minute warm-up, such as light cardio or dynamic stretching, to prepare your muscles and reduce the risk of injury.

o **Maintain Proper Technique**: Ensure correct form to maximize the effectiveness of your stretches and prevent injury. For static stretching, avoid bouncing and hold the stretch at a point of mild discomfort, not pain.

o **Breathe Deeply**: During stretching, breathe deeply and slowly to help relax your muscles and enhance the stretch. Proper breathing aids in achieving a deeper and more effective stretch.

o **Cool Down**: After your workout or flexibility session, incorporate gentle stretching or foam rolling to help relax your muscles and improve flexibility. This helps in recovery and maintains mobility.

Incorporating Flexibility Training into Your Routine

Integrate flexibility training with other exercise types—cardio, strength training, and balance work—for a comprehensive fitness routine. Aim to include flexibility exercises at least 2-3 times per week, focusing on different muscle groups and types of stretching. Regularly incorporating flexibility training helps maintain and improve range of motion and overall movement quality.

Flexibility training is crucial for enhancing mobility, reducing muscle tension, and supporting overall physical health. By understanding and correctly performing various flexibility exercises, you can build a well-rounded fitness routine that contributes to long-term movement efficiency and well-being.

Balance Training: Enhancing Stability and Coordination

Balance training is a fundamental component of a comprehensive fitness program, focusing on improving stability, coordination, and functional movement. It involves exercises that challenge your body's ability to maintain equilibrium, which is essential for everyday activities and injury prevention. Understanding the different types of balance exercises and how to perform them correctly is crucial for achieving a well-rounded and effective fitness routine.

What is Balance Training?

Balance training involves exercises designed to enhance your ability to maintain control of your body's position, whether stationary or in motion. These exercises target the core, legs, and stabilizing muscles, improving overall stability and coordination. Common balance exercises include standing on one leg, using balance boards, and performing stability ball exercises. The primary goal is to improve balance, reduce the risk of falls, and support functional fitness.

Types of Balance Exercises

- o **Static Balance Exercises**: Focus on maintaining a stable position without movement. Examples include standing on one leg or holding a pose on a balance board. These exercises enhance your ability to maintain balance while stationary.

- o **Dynamic Balance Exercises**: Involve maintaining balance while in motion. Activities like walking heel-to-toe, performing lunges, or stepping over obstacles improve your ability to balance during movement.

- o **Core Stability Exercises**: Target the muscles of the core to support overall balance and stability. Examples include planks, Russian twists, and stability ball rollouts. A strong core enhances your ability to maintain balance and control.

- o **Proprioceptive Training**: Uses equipment like balance pads, stability balls, or wobble boards to challenge your balance and coordination. These tools create an unstable surface that forces your body to adapt and stabilize.

How to Perform Balance Exercises Correctly

- o **Warm-Up**: Begin with a 5-10 minute warm-up, such as light cardio or dynamic stretching, to prepare your body and reduce the risk of injury.

- o **Maintain Proper Form**: Ensure correct posture and alignment to maximize the effectiveness of your balance exercises and prevent injury. For example, when performing a single-leg stand, keep your supporting knee slightly bent and your core engaged.

- o **Start with Basic Exercises**: If you're new to balance training, begin with simpler exercises and gradually progress to more challenging movements as your balance improves.

- o **Incorporate Breathing**: Focus on steady, controlled breathing to help maintain balance and relax your muscles. Proper breathing can enhance your stability and performance during exercises.

Incorporating Balance Training into Your Routine

To achieve a balanced fitness routine, integrate balance training with cardio, strength training, and flexibility exercises. Aim for at least 2-3 balance training sessions per week, incorporating various exercises to challenge different aspects of balance and stability. Regular practice helps improve coordination, reduce fall risk, and enhance overall functional fitness.

Balance training is crucial for improving stability, coordination, and overall movement quality. By understanding and correctly performing various balance exercises, you can build a well-rounded fitness routine that supports long-term health and functional ability.

In summary

Mastering cardio, strength, flexibility, and balance exercises is essential for a well-rounded fitness routine. Each type contributes uniquely to overall health, from boosting cardiovascular endurance and building muscle to enhancing mobility and stability. Understanding and integrating these exercises effectively ensures a balanced program that supports long-term fitness and well-being.

Workout Programs and Planning

An effective workout program should be designed around your specific fitness goals, whether they are strength building, endurance enhancement, weight loss, or a combination of these. Here's a brief overview of how to structure workouts for various objectives:

Strength Training

Strength training focuses on building muscle mass and improving overall strength. The primary components of a strength-focused workout include:

Exercises

Incorporate compound movements such as squats, deadlifts, bench presses, and pull-ups. These exercises engage multiple muscle groups and are effective for building overall strength.

Sets and Reps

Aim for 3-5 sets of 4-8 repetitions for heavy lifts to increase muscle strength. For muscle hypertrophy (growth), include 3-4 sets of 8-12 repetitions with moderate weights.

Rest Periods

Allow 1-2 minutes of rest between sets for heavy lifts and 30-60 seconds for lighter weights to maintain intensity.

Progression

Gradually increase the weight or resistance as you become stronger to continue challenging your muscles and making gains.

Endurance Training

Endurance training improves cardiovascular health and stamina. Key elements for endurance workouts include:

Exercises

Engage in aerobic activities such as running, cycling, swimming, or rowing. These exercises help improve cardiovascular fitness and overall stamina.

Duration and Intensity

Perform steady-state cardio for longer durations (30-60 minutes) at a moderate intensity. Incorporate interval training with high-intensity bursts followed by rest periods to enhance cardiovascular efficiency.

Frequency

Aim for at least 3-5 sessions per week, balancing longer, moderate-intensity sessions with shorter, high-intensity interval workouts.

Progression

Increase the duration or intensity of your workouts gradually to continue improving endurance and avoiding plateaus.

Weight Loss

A weight loss program combines cardiovascular and strength training to maximize calorie burn and muscle retention. Key components include:

Exercises

Mix aerobic exercises (e.g., running, cycling) with strength training (e.g., weight lifting, bodyweight exercises). This combination helps burn calories and preserve muscle mass.

Intensity and Duration

Use high-intensity interval training (HIIT) to maximize calorie burn in shorter timeframes. Include moderate-intensity cardio sessions for longer durations (30-45 minutes) to enhance overall calorie expenditure.

Frequency

Incorporate at least 3-4 cardio sessions and 2-3 strength training sessions per week. Ensure a balanced approach to avoid overtraining and promote effective fat loss.

Nutrition

Pair your exercise program with a balanced diet to support weight loss. Monitor calorie intake and focus on nutrient-dense foods to fuel your workouts and recovery.

Incorporating Principles of Progression and Recovery

Progression

Gradually increase the intensity, volume, or complexity of your workouts to continue making progress. This could mean adding more weight, increasing the duration of cardio sessions, or incorporating more challenging exercises. Progressive overload is key to improving strength and endurance over time.

Recovery

Allow adequate time for your muscles and body to recover between workouts. This includes incorporating rest days and ensuring you have a proper balance of exercise and recovery. Recovery is crucial for preventing overtraining, reducing injury risk, and allowing muscles to repair and grow stronger.

Designing Your Workout Plan

Creating an effective workout plan involves careful consideration of several key factors to ensure your routine is balanced, achievable, and aligned with your fitness goals. Here's a detailed look at how to design your workout plan:

Frequency

- o **Weekly Exercise Schedule:** Decide how many days per week you will dedicate to exercise. For a balanced routine, aim to incorporate different types of workouts throughout the week. A common recommendation is to exercise 4-6 days a week, depending on your fitness level and goals.
- o **Balance of Workouts:** Allocate time for each type of exercise, including cardio, strength, flexibility, and balance. For instance, if you plan to work out five days a week, you might include three days of cardio, one day of strength training, and one day of flexibility or balance work.
- o **Rest Days:** Integrate rest days into your schedule to allow your body to recover. Rest is crucial for muscle repair, preventing burnout, and reducing the risk of overtraining. Ensure at least one or two days of rest or active recovery per week.

Duration

- o **Workout Length:** Plan the length of each workout based on your fitness goals and schedule. For general fitness, aim for 30-60 minutes per session. Cardio sessions might be longer, while strength training sessions could be shorter but more intense.
- o **Alignment with Goals:** Adjust the duration of your workouts according to your objectives. For weight

loss, you might include longer cardio sessions, whereas strength training sessions might focus on shorter, high-intensity workouts with more focus on form and resistance.

- o **Time Management:** Ensure your workout duration fits into your daily schedule. Consistency is key, so it's important to choose a workout length that you can maintain over the long term without compromising other responsibilities.

Variety

- o **Exercise Mix:** Incorporate a variety of exercises to keep your routine engaging and prevent plateaus. Combining different types of workouts not only makes your routine more interesting but also ensures that you target various muscle groups and fitness aspects.
- o **Targeting Muscle Groups:** Include exercises that work different muscle groups to achieve balanced muscle development. For example, alternate between upper body, lower body, and core exercises throughout the week.
- o **Preventing Monotony:** Regularly change up your exercises to keep your routine fresh and challenging. This might involve trying new activities, adjusting the intensity, or varying your workout formats (e.g., switching from steady-state cardio to interval training).

Flexibility and Adaptation

- o **Adjusting the Plan:** Be prepared to modify your workout plan based on your progress, feedback from your body, or changes in your schedule. Flexibility in

> your plan allows you to adapt to evolving fitness levels, goals, or life circumstances.
> - **Listening to Your Body:** Pay attention to how your body responds to different workouts. Adjust frequency, duration, or exercise types as needed to avoid overtraining and ensure that you're meeting your fitness goals effectively.

Tracking and Evaluation

> - **Progress Monitoring:** Regularly track your progress to evaluate the effectiveness of your workout plan. Use fitness assessments, personal records, or subjective measures (e.g., how you feel) to gauge improvements and make necessary adjustments.
> - **Goal Setting:** Set short-term and long-term goals to stay motivated and focused. Regularly review and update these goals based on your progress and any changes in your fitness journey.

By carefully considering frequency, duration, and variety, and allowing for flexibility and regular evaluation, you can design a workout plan that is both effective and sustainable. This thoughtful approach helps ensure that your fitness routine supports your goals, maintains engagement, and promotes overall well-being.

Monitoring and Adjusting

Regularly assess your progress and adjust your program as needed. This might involve increasing weights, altering workout intensity, or changing exercises to avoid plateaus and keep your routine effective.

In summary

Designing an effective workout program requires understanding how to structure workouts for your specific goals, applying principles of progression, and incorporating adequate recovery. By following these guidelines, you can create a well-rounded fitness plan that helps you achieve your objectives while minimizing the risk of injury and overtraining.

Nutrition and Hydration

Proper nutrition and hydration are critical components of a successful fitness regimen. Understanding how to effectively fuel your body with the right nutrients and fluids is essential for optimizing physical performance, supporting recovery, and promoting overall health. Here's a detailed overview of how to approach nutrition and hydration to enhance your fitness journey:

Nutrition

Macronutrients

The three primary macronutrients—carbohydrates, proteins, and fats—play distinct roles in supporting fitness goals.

- o **Carbohydrates**: Provide the primary source of energy for exercise, especially for high-intensity and endurance activities. Focus on complex carbs like whole grains, fruits, and vegetables for sustained energy.

- o **Proteins**: Crucial for muscle repair and growth. Include lean protein sources such as chicken, fish, tofu, and legumes to support muscle recovery and development.

- o **Fats**: Essential for overall health and energy. Incorporate healthy fats from sources like avocados, nuts, seeds, and olive oil to support cell function and hormone production.

Micronutrients

Vitamins and minerals are vital for various bodily functions, including energy production, immune support, and muscle contraction. Ensure a balanced intake of micronutrients by consuming a variety of fruits, vegetables, and whole foods.

Timing and Balance

- o **Pre-Workout Nutrition**: Consume a balanced meal or snack 1-3 hours before exercise to fuel your workout. Focus on a combination of carbs and protein to optimize energy and muscle function.

- o **Post-Workout Nutrition**: Replenish energy stores and support muscle recovery with a post-workout meal or snack containing carbs and protein. Aim to eat within 30-60 minutes after exercise to maximize recovery benefits.

Hydration

Importance of Hydration

Proper hydration is essential for maintaining performance, regulating body temperature, and facilitating nutrient transport. Dehydration can impair exercise performance and recovery, so it's crucial to stay adequately hydrated.

Fluid Intake Recommendations

- o **Daily Hydration**: Aim for about 8-10 cups (2-2.5 liters) of water per day, though individual needs may vary based on activity level, climate, and body size.

- o **Pre-Exercise Hydration**: Drink water before workouts to ensure your body starts off well-hydrated. A good rule of thumb is to drink 16-20 ounces (500-600 ml) of water 1-2 hours before exercise.

o **During Exercise**: Sip water regularly during exercise, especially for workouts lasting longer than 30 minutes or in hot conditions. Aim to drink about 7-10 ounces (200-300 ml) every 15-20 minutes.

Hydration Strategies

o **Electrolytes:** For prolonged or intense exercise, consider beverages with electrolytes (sodium, potassium) to replace lost minerals. Sports drinks or electrolyte tablets can be beneficial for maintaining electrolyte balance.

o **Monitoring Hydration:** Pay attention to signs of dehydration, such as dark urine or feeling excessively thirsty. Adjust fluid intake based on your individual needs and exercise conditions.

Balancing Nutrition and Hydration

Personalized Plan

Creating a personalized nutrition and hydration plan is essential for optimizing your fitness results and overall health. Here's how to tailor your approach:

o **Assess Your Goals**: Start by defining your specific fitness objectives, whether it's building muscle, improving endurance, or losing weight. Your nutritional and hydration needs will vary based on these goals. For example, a muscle-building plan might focus on higher protein intake, while a weight loss plan might emphasize calorie control.

o **Evaluate Your Activity Level**: Your daily activity level greatly influences your nutritional and hydration needs. Sedentary individuals will have different requirements compared to those who engage in regular intense exercise.

Adjust your calorie intake and hydration strategies to align with your activity level to ensure you're meeting your energy and recovery needs.

o **Consider Dietary Preferences**: Tailor your plan to fit your dietary preferences and restrictions. Whether you follow a vegetarian, vegan, or specific dietary regimen, ensure your nutrition plan provides adequate nutrients to support your fitness goals. For instance, vegetarians might need to focus on alternative protein sources such as legumes and soy products.

o **Seek Professional Guidance**: Consulting with a registered dietitian or nutritionist can provide personalized advice and meal planning tailored to your needs. These professionals can help design a plan that aligns with your fitness goals, dietary preferences, and any medical conditions, ensuring a comprehensive and balanced approach.

Consistency and Adaptation

Maintaining a consistent approach to nutrition and hydration is key for achieving and sustaining fitness progress. Here's how to ensure long-term success:

o **Routine Adherence**: Consistency in your eating and hydration habits helps support continuous progress. Stick to your meal plan and hydration schedule, making it a regular part of your daily routine. This consistency is crucial for seeing long-term benefits and achieving your fitness goals.

o **Adapt to Changes**: Be prepared to adjust your nutrition and hydration plan based on changes in your exercise routine, goals, or personal circumstances. For instance, if you increase workout intensity or duration, you may need to adjust your calorie intake or hydration strategies to accommodate these changes.

o **Responsive Adjustments**: Pay attention to how your body responds to different aspects of your plan. If you notice changes in energy levels, performance, or recovery, make necessary adjustments. Adapt your plan based on these observations to maintain optimal effectiveness and support your evolving fitness needs.

Tracking and Evaluation

Monitoring and evaluating your nutrition and hydration practices are essential for ensuring they support your fitness goals and overall health. Here's how to effectively track and assess your progress:

Monitoring Intake

Use tools such as food diaries, mobile apps, or wearable technology to track your daily food and fluid intake. Monitoring helps ensure you are meeting your nutritional and hydration goals. Apps can provide detailed insights into your macro and micronutrient intake, helping you make informed decisions about your diet.

Evaluate Impact

Regularly assess how your nutrition and hydration practices affect your performance, recovery, and general well-being. Track changes in energy levels, workout performance, and overall health to evaluate the impact of your dietary and hydration strategies. Adjust your plan based on this evaluation to optimize your fitness results and ensure continued progress.

In summary

Proper nutrition and hydration are crucial for enhancing workout effectiveness, supporting recovery, and maintaining overall health.

By creating a personalized plan, maintaining consistency, adapting as needed, and effectively tracking and evaluating your practices, you can fuel your body effectively and achieve your fitness goals. Understanding and applying these principles will help you make informed choices, support your fitness journey, and promote long-term health and well-being.

Injury Prevention and Management

Injury prevention and management are crucial for maintaining a safe and effective fitness routine. Understanding how to prevent injuries and address them when they occur helps ensure a sustainable and enjoyable fitness journey. This chapter provides a comprehensive overview of how to approach injury prevention and management to support long-term fitness success.

Injury Prevention

Proper Exercise Form

- **Learn Proper Techniques**: Correct exercise form is fundamental to avoiding injuries. Poor technique can lead to strain and misalignment, increasing the risk of injury. For example, during exercises like squats or deadlifts, maintaining proper posture and alignment is essential to prevent lower back injuries. Proper form ensures that exercises target the intended muscle groups effectively and safely.

- **Seek Professional Guidance**: Working with a certified personal trainer or coach can provide valuable feedback and guidance on your exercise form. Trainers can demonstrate correct techniques, identify and correct mistakes, and tailor instructions to your individual needs. This personalized feedback helps you build a solid foundation for safe and effective exercise.

Warm-Up

- **Dynamic Warm-Up**: A well-structured warm-up is essential for preparing your body for exercise and reducing the risk of injury. Dynamic warm-ups involve movements that increase your heart rate and prepare your muscles and joints for more intense activity. Activities like high knees, butt kicks, and arm swings help increase blood flow to your muscles, improve flexibility, and enhance overall readiness for exercise.

- o **Targeted Warm-Up**: Focus your warm-up on the muscle groups you plan to work during your session. For example, if your workout includes leg exercises, perform warm-up exercises that engage your lower body, such as leg swings or lunges. This targeted approach ensures that the specific muscles and joints used in your workout are adequately prepared.

Cool-Down

- o **Gradual Decrease**: Cooling down after exercise helps your body transition back to a resting state and reduces the risk of post-workout soreness. Gradually decreasing the intensity of your activity allows your heart rate and breathing to return to normal. Activities like light jogging or walking are effective for this purpose.

- o **Static Stretching**: Incorporate static stretching into your cool-down routine to help relax your muscles and improve flexibility. Static stretches involve holding a stretch for 15-30 seconds and can help alleviate muscle tightness and improve overall flexibility. Stretching major muscle groups that were worked during your session can also aid in reducing muscle soreness and promoting recovery.

Managing Common Injuries

Recognize Common Injuries

- **Sprains and Strains**: Sprains and strains are common injuries that result from overstretching or sudden movements. Sprains involve the stretching or tearing of ligaments, while strains affect muscles or tendons. Symptoms may include pain, swelling, bruising, and difficulty moving the affected area.

- **Tendinitis**: Tendinitis is inflammation of a tendon, often caused by repetitive stress or overuse. Commonly affected areas include the knees (patellar tendinitis), shoulders (rotator cuff tendinitis), and elbows (tennis elbow). Symptoms typically include pain, swelling, and tenderness in the affected tendon.

Immediate Response

- **R.I.C.E. Method**: The R.I.C.E. method—Rest, Ice, Compression, and Elevation—is a standard approach for managing acute injuries. Rest the affected area to prevent further strain. Apply ice for 15-20 minutes several times a day to reduce swelling and pain. Use compression, such as an elastic bandage, to minimize swelling. Elevate the injured area above heart level to reduce blood flow and swelling.

- **Seek Medical Attention**: If symptoms persist, worsen, or are accompanied by severe pain, loss of function, or visible deformity, seek medical attention. A healthcare professional can provide an accurate diagnosis, prescribe appropriate treatment, and offer guidance on rehabilitation and recovery.

Rehabilitation and Recovery

- o **Follow a Rehab Program**: Adhering to a prescribed rehabilitation program is essential for effective recovery. A physical therapist can design a program that includes exercises to strengthen the injured area, improve flexibility, and restore function. Following the program diligently helps ensure a full recovery and reduces the risk of re-injury.

- o **Gradual Return to Exercise**: Once cleared by a healthcare professional, reintroduce exercise gradually. Start with low-impact activities and gradually increase intensity based on your comfort and healing progress. Avoid jumping back into high-intensity workouts too soon, as this can exacerbate the injury or lead to further complications.

Long-Term Injury Prevention

Strength and Flexibility

- o **Incorporate Strength Training**: Building strength in key muscle groups supports joint stability and reduces the risk of injury. Strength training exercises, such as resistance training or bodyweight exercises, help improve muscle balance and support overall functional movement.

- o **Include Flexibility Exercises**: Regular flexibility exercises enhance joint range of motion and reduce muscle tightness. Incorporate activities like yoga or dynamic stretching into your routine to maintain and improve flexibility, which can help prevent injuries and enhance overall mobility.

Listen to Your Body

- **Recognize Warning Signs**: Pay attention to signs of discomfort or pain during or after exercise. Persistent or unusual soreness, sharp pain, or swelling are indicators that you may need to adjust your workout or seek medical advice. Listening to your body helps prevent overtraining and reduces the risk of injuries.

- **Adjust Workouts as Needed**: Modify your exercise routine based on how your body feels. If you experience discomfort or pain, consider reducing the intensity or altering exercises to avoid exacerbating the issue. Making adjustments based on feedback from your body helps ensure a safe and effective fitness routine.

Consistent Maintenance

- **Review and Adjust**: Regularly review and adjust your exercise techniques and routines to ensure they align with your fitness goals and physical condition. As you progress in your fitness journey, periodically assess your routines to address any potential risks or areas for improvement.

- **Preventive Measures**: Adopt preventive measures, such as proper warm-up and cool-down practices, consistent strength and flexibility training, and mindful exercise techniques, to support long-term fitness and minimize injury risk.

In Summary

Effective injury prevention and management are crucial for maintaining a safe and successful fitness routine. By focusing on proper exercise form, incorporating effective warm-up and cool-down practices, and understanding how to address common injuries, you can reduce the risk of injury and support your long-term fitness journey. Adopting a proactive approach to injury prevention, managing injuries effectively, and maintaining consistent practices will help you achieve your fitness goals while safeguarding your health and well-being.

Motivation and Mental Health

Maintaining motivation and addressing mental health are fundamental for achieving and sustaining long-term success in fitness. This chapter delves into the intricate relationship between motivation, mental health, and fitness, offering practical strategies for overcoming obstacles, setting meaningful goals, and fostering a supportive mindset. We will explore how to integrate these elements into a cohesive approach for a well-rounded and successful fitness journey.

The Essence of Motivation in Fitness

Motivation acts as the driving force behind your commitment to fitness. It influences your consistency, effort, and overall engagement with your fitness routine. To build and sustain motivation, consider the following:

Intrinsic vs. Extrinsic Motivation

- **Intrinsic Motivation**: This stems from internal desires such as personal satisfaction, a sense of achievement, or the enjoyment of exercise itself. Cultivate intrinsic motivation by setting personal milestones and focusing on how exercise makes you feel better physically and mentally.

- **Extrinsic Motivation**: This involves external rewards such as praise, recognition, or tangible rewards. While it can provide initial motivation, it's essential to balance it with intrinsic goals for sustained engagement. Use extrinsic rewards as occasional incentives rather than primary motivators.

Effective Goal Setting

- **SMART Goals**: Create goals that are Specific, Measurable, Achievable, Relevant, and Time-bound. For example, "Increase my bench press by 20 pounds in three months" provides clear targets and a timeline, making it easier to track progress and stay motivated.

- **Short-Term vs. Long-Term Goals**: Break long-term goals into smaller, short-term objectives to maintain motivation and provide regular feedback on your progress. Achieving short-term goals builds confidence and keeps you focused on the bigger picture.

Monitoring and Tracking Progress

- **Journaling**: Keep a fitness journal to document workouts, progress, and personal reflections. Journals help track improvements, recognize patterns, and maintain a record of achievements.

- **Fitness Apps and Wearables**: Utilize technology such as fitness apps or wearables to monitor your performance, set reminders, and analyze data. These tools provide real-time feedback and can help keep you accountable.

Reward Systems and Celebrations

- **Incorporate Rewards**: Develop a reward system for achieving milestones. Rewards could be non-food-related, such as a new workout outfit, a massage, or a day off. Rewards reinforce positive behavior and celebrate progress.

- **Celebrate Achievements**: Take time to acknowledge and celebrate both small and significant achievements. Celebrations reinforce positive behaviors and remind you of the progress made.

Overcoming Setbacks and Plateaus

- **Reframe Setbacks**: View setbacks as opportunities to learn and grow rather than failures. Analyze what led to the setback, adjust your plan, and use the experience to strengthen your resilience.

- **Addressing Plateaus**: If you hit a plateau, consider modifying your routine or trying new activities to reinvigorate your interest and challenge your body in different ways.

Addressing Mental Health in Fitness

Mental health significantly impacts your fitness journey, influencing motivation, energy levels, and overall well-being. Here's how to address mental health to enhance your fitness progress:

The Psychological Benefits of Exercise

- **Mood Improvement**: Exercise triggers the release of endorphins, which are natural mood lifters. Regular physical activity can help alleviate symptoms of depression and anxiety, contributing to improved mental health.

- **Stress Reduction**: Physical activity reduces stress hormones like cortisol and promotes relaxation. Incorporate exercises known for their calming effects, such as yoga or swimming, to manage stress effectively.

Stress Management Techniques

- **Mindfulness and Meditation**: Practice mindfulness and meditation to reduce stress and improve mental clarity. These techniques help you stay present and manage anxiety, enhancing your overall well-being.

- **Deep Breathing Exercises**: Implement deep breathing exercises to calm your nervous system and reduce stress. Techniques such as diaphragmatic breathing can help you relax before or after workouts.

Seeking Professional Support

- **Therapy and Counseling**: If you face persistent mental health challenges, consult a mental health professional. Therapy can provide strategies for managing mental health issues and offer support during your fitness journey.

- **Support Groups**: Join support groups or online communities where you can share experiences and receive encouragement from others facing similar challenges.

Integrating Self-Care Practices

- **Balancing Work and Life**: Ensure that fitness does not become a source of additional stress. Maintain a balance between your workout routine and other life responsibilities to prevent burnout.

- **Engaging in Enjoyable Activities**: Incorporate hobbies and activities that you enjoy outside of fitness. Engaging in pleasurable activities enhances overall happiness and contributes to a positive mindset.

Cultivating a Positive Mindset

A positive mindset enhances your ability to stay motivated and committed to your fitness goals. Here's how to develop and maintain a positive outlook:

Positive Self-Talk and Affirmations

- **Challenge Negative Thoughts**: Replace self-criticism with positive affirmations. Practice self-compassion and focus on what you are doing well rather than dwelling on perceived shortcomings.

- **Affirmation Practices**: Use affirmations to reinforce your goals and boost self-confidence. For example, "I am strong and capable of achieving my fitness goals" can help maintain a positive outlook.

Building Resilience and Adaptability

- **Develop Coping Strategies**: Learn coping strategies for dealing with setbacks and challenges. Techniques such as problem-solving and adapting your goals can enhance resilience and help you stay on track.

- **Embrace a Growth Mindset**: Cultivate a growth mindset by viewing challenges as opportunities to learn and grow. Embrace change and view failures as stepping stones to success.

Creating a Supportive Environment

- **Build a Support Network**: Surround yourself with people who support and motivate you. Whether it's friends, family, or workout partners, a supportive network can provide encouragement and accountability.

- o **Participate in Fitness Communities**: Engage with fitness communities or groups to find camaraderie and motivation. Being part of a community provides social support and shared experiences.

Finding Enjoyment in Fitness

- o **Explore Different Activities**: Try various forms of exercise to find what you enjoy most. Experiment with different classes, sports, or outdoor activities to keep your routine engaging and enjoyable.

- o **Focus on Fun**: Shift your focus from purely achieving goals to enjoying the process. Find ways to make workouts fun and rewarding to sustain long-term interest and motivation.

Integrating Motivation and Mental Health into Your Fitness Routine

For a successful fitness journey, integrate motivation and mental health strategies into your routine. Regularly assess your mental well-being, adjust your motivational techniques as needed, and ensure a holistic approach that supports both physical and psychological health.

Regular Reflection and Adjustment

- o **Self-Assessment**: Periodically evaluate your motivation levels and mental health. Reflect on what's working well and what might need adjustment to stay aligned with your goals.

- o **Flexible Planning**: Adapt your fitness plan based on your evolving needs and circumstances. Being flexible helps maintain motivation and prevents feelings of frustration.

Creating a Balanced Routine

- o **Combine Activities**: Integrate various fitness activities to keep your routine diverse and engaging. Balance cardio, strength training, flexibility, and balance exercises to support overall health and prevent boredom.

- o **Prioritize Mental and Physical Health**: Ensure that your fitness routine supports both mental and physical health. Make adjustments to prioritize mental well-being alongside achieving physical fitness goals.

In summary

Motivation and mental health are integral to achieving and maintaining long-term success in fitness. By understanding and implementing strategies to enhance motivation, address mental health, and cultivate a positive mindset, you lay a strong foundation for a fulfilling and sustainable fitness journey. Integrate these principles into your routine to ensure comprehensive progress and overall well-being.

ABOUT THE AUTHOR

Anila Ferrero | Author | Investor | Entrepreneur